DIET

COACH

All the advice you need to succeed at weight loss

and keep the weight off

KIMBERLY WILLIS

piatkus

PIATKUS

First published in the US in 2011 by Atria Books
as *The Little Book of Diet Help*
First published in Great Britain in 2012 by Piatkus
as *The Little Book of Diet Help*
This paperback edition published in 2013 by Piatkus

Disclaimer: this book is not a substitute for proper medical advice.
If you believe you are in need of medical interventions, please see a
medical practitioner as soon as possible. The author and publisher
cannot accept any responsibility for illness or injury arising
out of failure to seek professional medical advice
from a qualified medical practitioner.

A CIP catalogue record for this book
is available from the British Library.

ISBN 978-0-7499-5701-8

Designed by Sam Charrington
Printed and bound in Great Britain by
Clays Ltd, St Ives plc

Papers used by Piatkus are from well-managed forests
and other responsible sources.

MIX
Paper from
responsible sources
FSC
www.fsc.org   FSC® C104740

Piatkus
An imprint of
Little, Brown Book Group
100 Victoria Embankment
London EC4Y 0DY

An Hachette UK Company
www.hachette.co.uk

www.piatkus.co.uk

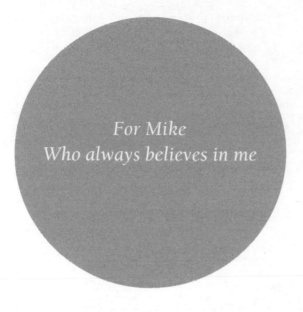

For Mike
Who always believes in me

Contents

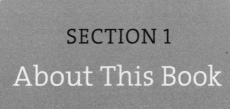

SECTION 1

About This Book

So You Want to Lose Weight . . .

This isn't just another diet book. This book is different.

You already know what you need to do to lose weight.

This book will take you on a journey that will help shift the emotional blocks that have been stopping you from becoming your slimmer self so that you can start making the choices in your life which will give you the body you deserve.

I will help you take control of your life, to shed that unwanted weight so that you become the best version of yourself.

This book will give you some knowledge about food and how it affects you. As a result, you will find that you naturally begin to make changes to what you put into your body.

The way this book differs from other weight-loss methods is that I will help you to adjust your attitudes to yourself, your body and food by using exercises derived from yoga, acupressure, hypnotherapy and neuro-linguistic programming.

These therapies are widely used around the world to help individuals deal with a variety of issues, from irrational anxieties to confidence boosting. You will find that by changing your thought patterns, your behaviour will change – and when you reinforce those new, positive behaviours, you will start to free yourself of your negative habits, helping you to lose weight more easily and more permanently.

All the exercises in this book are ones that I have successfully used with my weight-loss groups. Individuals in those groups have found that through these exercises they were able to change their habits, feel more positive, more motivated and, ultimately, lose weight more easily than when they had been on a restrictive diet.

Who am I? – I am a weight-loss specialist and for many years I have worked with individuals and groups helping them become naturally slimmer, healthier and happier with their bodies.

Most importantly, I am now here to help you. Today is the first day of the new you.

Kimberly Willis

How should you use this book?

I would suggest that you read through the whole book initially, getting a feel for how it is laid out.

Try some of the exercises and tips to see what works for you. Start to incorporate them into your day.

When using the tapping techniques (see pages 7–8) give yourself some quiet time, away from everyone else where you can really focus on your thoughts and how you are feeling.

You might find that you want to have this book with you during the day so that you can refer to it when a craving strikes and remind yourself of the useful hints and tips.

Note: The emotional work in this book can sometimes uncover deep-seated issues; if you find that this is the case for you I would suggest you seek professional help from a registered therapist or counsellor.

Your aim is:

- To feel positive about yourself, your body and how you look.
- To eat when you are hungry.
- To stop eating when you are no longer hungry.
- To free yourself from cravings.
- To feel motivated to exercise more.
- To lose weight easily and naturally.

What is keeping you attached to that excess weight?

If you are reading this book you have probably tried many diets (otherwise why would you have picked it up?).

Your past has emotional chains around you.

These chains stop you from moving forward.

They keep you attached to that excess weight.

Break these chains and you will find that you can let go of the weight you no longer need.

Working through the exercises in this book will help free you from the chains tying you to the past.

You will tap into your negative emotions by accessing powerful acupressure points. This will help break down the hold that these emotions have over you.

Tapping explained

Within this book, you will find a number of 'tapping' exercises, which are carried out on acupressure points throughout your body.

Some of these exercises are derived from EFT (emotional freedom technique), developed by Gary Craig, which uses a specific set of acupressure points.

The theory behind these techniques is that all emotional upsets are caused by disturbances in the body's energy system. Therefore, if you correct the energy disturbance, the emotional upset will disappear.

This is a very ancient practice, with deep historical roots. Around five thousand years ago, the Chinese discovered that pressing certain points on the body could help reduce pain. Using this knowledge, the Chinese went on to plot the energy lines of the body, known

⟶

today as meridians. From this, the fields of acupressure and acupuncture were born.

Since then, the existence of energy lines within the body have been widely discussed and accepted as a tenet of many wellness therapies. Gently tapping along these meridians – while focusing on the issue that is bothering you – helps shift the energy in your body, settling the disturbances that are causing negative emotions to flare.

As a therapist I have seen at first hand how these techniques can result in amazing changes.

After using one of the tapping exercises you may notice an instant change in how you feel – or, after a few days, you may look back over your recent behaviour and realise that there has indeed been a positive shift in your actions.

Creating Change

When you come across something that is an issue for you, like negative beliefs or food cravings, follow the tapping guide, repeating the phrases for that issue (see pages 55–6, 115–16, 160–1 and 182–3). Wait a week, then repeat. This will create positive change.

YOUR TAPPING MAP

When tapping to break down negative emotions, follow the points on the diagram on the next page and tap each point with your index and middle fingers about eight times, saying a negative statement (see page 54 for examples) as you tap.

- **Begin by tapping your Karate Chop point, which is located on the side of your hand below your little finger, a soft fleshy area between your finger and wrist bone. If you were actually doing a karate chop, this is the place your hand would hit the board.**

- **Move onto the Inner Eyebrow point (1), then the Outer Eyebrow point (2). Follow all the points on the face, continuing to repeat the statement. Follow the order that the points are numbered in.**

→

- Now place your arm diagonally across your chest so that your fingers rest on your collarbone and tap this point (6).

- Now you are ready to move onto the points on your hand. Using the opposite hand, tap on the side of each finger, next to the nail.

- Continue to the Gamut point. This is located on the top of your hand, in the 'V' that's created where the bones of your fourth and fifth fingers meet. Rub the skin in this 'V' gently.

- At the end of the sequence finish off by once again tapping the Karate Chop point.

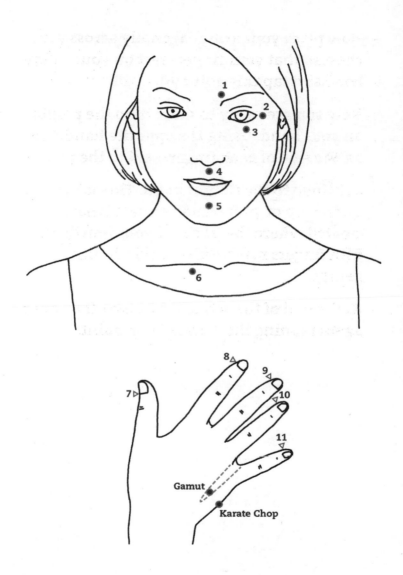

Neuro-linguistic programming (NLP)

This is a very complicated way of describing some of the easy techniques that are in this book. Really it is about language, how we use it and how it affects us. It is also about our feelings and behaviour.

NLP was developed by John Grinder and Richard Bandler in California in the 1970s. It uses language to help you shift your views and beliefs.

You'll see it put into action in some of the easy techniques that are in this book.

For example, if you alter the tone of your voice as you repeat an affirmation (see page 74), it can affect the way that you feel.

Or the way that you phrase something can affect your view of it:

'I am trying to lose weight, but it's hard.'
Becomes:
'I am losing weight easily each and every day.'

In both of these cases neuro-linguistic programming is at work.

NLP can help you shift to a new viewpoint to make you feel stronger and more positive about achieving your goal.

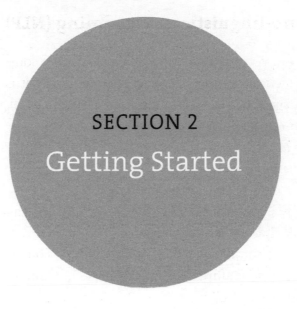

SECTION 2

Getting Started

When I begin with a new weight loss group everyone is sitting round nervously waiting for the course to start.

What do I do?

I get them to stand up and to start learning about their body: action first – both physical and emotional.

QUICK METABOLISM BOOSTER

- **Stand up.**

- **Place one hand on your stomach.**

- **Breathe deeply and slowly, through your nose, as if you could breathe into the depths of your stomach.**

- **Repeat for five breaths.**

Deep belly breathing boosts your metabolism – and when your metabolism is boosted, you burn more calories.

Remember:

Zero fat

Does not mean

Zero calories

Calories matter!

Feeling hungry?

Before reaching for a snack have a glass of water.

When you are thirsty your body can send out hunger signals, because it knows that you can get water from food.

Drink some water and you might find that your hunger disappears.

Q: How can you burn more calories watching TV at night?

A: Exercise in the morning!

This will boost your metabolism for the rest of the day.

Even when you are sitting in front of the TV in the evening you will be burning more calories than normal.

UNWANTED FOOD CRAVING?

Rub the area between your nose and your top lip with your first finger for about a minute.

This is a soothing point that will comfort you and reduce your craving.

Hug someone!

When you hug someone you feel better.

When you feel better you eat better.

So go on, have a cuddle.

THE TEMPTATION BATTLE

Sometimes it feels like a battle is going on in your mind. A part of you knows you are not hungry and really don't want that biscuit – but the other part of you is trying to convince yourself that it's OK to eat it – that after all, you deserve it.

Win the temptation battle!

If you find yourself tempted by snack food – like a bag of crisps, a bar of chocolate, or a late-night bowl of ice cream – try this exercise:

Touch the front part of your ear, that bit of cartilage that sticks out in front of your ear canal. Now, rub this between your thumb and first finger for a few minutes.

This is a strong acupressure point. It will help turn off cravings by redirecting your energy and lowering your appetite.

The chemicals at work in your body – insulin

Insulin is a hormone produced by your body, which allows it to absorb sugar. Here's how it works:

- Insulin is produced by the pancreas to absorb sugar from your bloodstream.

- Without insulin, your body cannot absorb and use this sugar.

- Sugar levels usually increase after a meal and as a result, insulin is produced.

The white refined carbohydrates and sugar hunger trap

Imagine a small child who has just eaten a huge bag of sweets. You know what happens next – his energy will be through the roof, and you'll practically have to peel him off the ceiling! Then before you know it, he'll crash – and he'll be irritable, unhappy, and likely to throw a tantrum. The same thing happens to adults when we eat processed foods – only instead of having a tantrum, we reach for more comfort foods. Here's how the chemistry works:

When you eat a bowl of pasta or a slice of cake…

- Your blood sugar zooms up.

- Your body releases more and more insulin to cope with the sudden increase.

- This excess insulin now causes your blood sugar levels to plummet.

- As a result you feel hungry, tired and irritable.

- You crave more food.

- You gain weight.

- More importantly, the rapid changes in sugar levels can result in insulin resistance which can lead to type 2 diabetes.

See 'Increased consumption of refined carbohydrates and the epidemic of type 2 diabetes in the United States: an ecologic assessment', by Lee S. Gross, Li Li, Earl S. Ford and Simin Liu, *American Journal of Clinical Nutrition*, Vol. 79, No. 5, 774–779, May 2004.

How can you stabilise your blood sugar?

Eating protein (eggs, turkey, chicken) or unrefined carbohydrates (that's brown pasta, brown rice and wheat or multigrain bread) prevents your blood sugar levels from spiking then plummeting, because their energy is released more slowly into your system causing a gradual rise in blood sugar levels.

When you stabilise your blood sugar:

- You feel fuller for longer.

- You will eat less.

- You will have more energy.

- You feel happier.

- You naturally lose weight.

Slim people stop eating when they are no longer hungry.

Overweight people stop eating when they are full.

AFTERNOON ENERGY BOOST

It's 4 p.m. You are tired and you need an energy boost.

Try this exercise as an alternative to going to the vending machine.

- **Stand up.**

- **Start marching, lifting your knees high and swinging the opposite arms.**

- **Now change to marching with the same arms and legs moving together.**

- **Repeat for a minute or two.**

Beware, beware the Bliss Point . . .

This is a special point in your brain that is stimulated by foods containing excessive amounts of **fat, salt and sugar**.

Think pizzas, biscuits and battered chicken.

Your brain loves it when this point is stimulated – it's like a drug and your brain doesn't want this feeling to end.

Part of your brain is going to try and keep you eating more and more of this food.

Even if you are full – stuffed – it will want you to eat more.

When the Bliss Point takes over you just can't stop eating. You are out of control.

If you recognise this behaviour then you need to avoid the foods that cause it.

Be aware of the foods that trigger this for you – this is what some manufacturers work towards. They want you to crave more and more of their product. Check the food labels for hidden salt, fat and sugar. Avoid these foods – they will beat any willpower!

As discussed in the excellent book *The End of Overeating* by David A. Kessler, Penguin, 2010.

Is all hunger the same?

Physical Hunger Comes hours after your last meal, this is a real hunger – one that you need to pay attention to.

Emotional Hunger Is caused by a negative or positive emotional trigger and can hit you at any time of the day, even if you have just eaten. *This type of hunger makes you gain weight.*

POSITIVE MIND AND BODY BOOST

This exercise will help you to feel good and to reconnect with your body.

- **Stand up.**

- **Bring your hands up in front of your chest in prayer position. As you inhale deeply, raise your hands, still in prayer position, above your head and look up.**

- **Hold this position as you inhale and exhale deeply for a couple of breaths. On your next out breath, bring your hands back in front of your chest. Repeat three times.**

- **Each time you raise your hands, feel yourself rooting into the ground as you simultaneously stretch towards the sky.**

- **Finish by tapping the top of your head with your fingertips, like raindrops. Notice how much calmer and lighter you feel.**

As you go about your day, periodically tune into your body, and recall the sensation of peace and ease that you felt as you finished this exercise.

Remember: When you feel better you eat better.

Eat better

Forget about eating right

Eating better is easier than eating right.

Eating right all the time can be hard work and depressing. Plus, you will probably fail – and when you do, you will then feel that much worse.

You can **succeed** at **eating better** than you have before. You can feel good about yourself and the positive changes that you are making.

When you fail at eating right, you will feel bad. When you feel bad you are more likely to comfort eat. This is what restrictive diets do to you.

Eating better makes you feel good. It's about the many small accomplishments that add up to a big change. Most importantly it allows you to be human – and humans make mistakes!

As discussed in *Mindless Eating* by Brian Wansink, Hay House, 2009.

Eat slowly!

Chew slowly!

Pay attention to what you are eating.

Binge eaters don't taste
what they are eating.

Notice your food. Smell
your food.

Chew slowly. Savour the tastes and
textures of each mouthful.

Appreciate your food.

Eat mindfully at the table,
not mindlessly in front
of the TV.

Stop forbidding certain foods

Why should you?? Try this:

Don't think of pink elephants.

I'll bet you did!

Now say to yourself 'I'm not having chocolate, no chocolate, no chocolate.'

What does your brain hear?

Chocolate Chocolate Chocolate
Chocolate Chocolate

This will beat even the strongest willpower.

Now you end up eating a kilo of chocolate.

So allow yourself a bit of chocolate and open up your thoughts and your energy for other, better things.

Allow yourself to be free of a restrictive diet.

Are you hungry?

Put your hand on your stomach and just notice how your stomach is really feeling.

Ignoring real physical hunger until you are starving causes your body to slow down as it thinks there is a famine and it must save energy.

When this happens, you stop burning calories.

Then – when you do eat, your body is worried that this might be all the food there is and it will store reserves (on your stomach and butt) and make you eat extra, just in case there is another famine on the way.

So when you are hungry – EAT!

Place your hand on your stomach once an hour just to check how it is feeling.

You have probably been ignoring your stomach for years – it could do with a bit of attention.

Eat slowly

Eat with awareness

Stop eating when you are no longer hungry

Feel that excess weight melt away

… It really is that simple

Are all calories the same?

NO!

Rate at which food leaves your stomach:

- **Protein:** at around four calories per minute.
- **Sugar and Carbohydrates:** at up to 30 calories per minute.

This means:

Eating high protein foods will keep you fuller for longer as they are in your stomach for longer.

As a result, you will eat less and lose more weight.

The chemicals at work in your body – serotonin

Serotonin is a chemical in the brain and is responsible for your 'happy feeling'. It also helps regulate moods, helping you to feel calmer and to sleep well. But it also exists in large quantities in the gut. There is a complex relationship between the stomach and the brain, which makes it very important to look after your body's serotonin levels.

Low serotonin levels have been linked to feeling *emotionally* low.

Refined carbohydrates will result in a short-term boost in serotonin; but the pleasure this leads to will quickly disappear as your blood sugar levels rapidly drop, leaving you feeling tired and down and craving even more refined carbohydrates.

If dieting in the past has left you feeling melancholy or unhappy, it's probably because you weren't taking proper care of your serotonin levels. When you begin to change your diet it is important that you support your body with nutrients and a lifestyle that will promote both your physical and mental wellbeing.

Boost your serotonin levels and feel good

You can start by paying attention to the foods you are eating, as some contain tryptophan. Your body needs tryptophan in order to make serotonin, so there are literally some foods that can boost your mood and your energy.

Walnuts, turkey, chicken, fish, bananas and avocados do this. (Although they might not make the world's greatest smoothie!)

Also salmon, almonds, eggs and complex carbohydrates, like oatmeal or whole wheat.

Exercise, sleep and being with other people will also boost your serotonin levels.

Pets

Sunlight

Positive thoughts

These all make you feel better and, as a result, you will eat better – and be more motivated to look after your body.

Take care with aspartame

Aspartame could deplete your serotonin levels, causing you to feel down.

As a result, you might crave comfort foods and fall into the trap of emotional eating.

Since many low fat and low calorie foods contain aspartame, beware – some so called 'diet foods' can lead to weight gain.

See 'Direct and indirect cellular effects of aspartame on the brain' in P. Humphries, E. Pretorius, H. Naude, *European Journal of Clinical Nutrition*, Vol. 62, 451–462, 2008.

Protein stabilises blood sugar, reduces your appetite and will reduce the amount of food you eat in a day.

Good sources of protein include: grilled chicken, eggs, beans, fish, tofu, almonds, pumpkin seeds, beans.

Listen Listen Listen

Listen to your body: when it is physically hungry – eat.

Choose something good for your body.

Your body will believe that there is plenty of food and your metabolism will speed up.

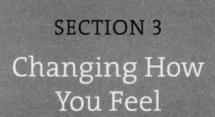

SECTION 3

Changing How
You Feel

It's cold, grey and raining outside. The cat has been sick in the hallway. You are having a bad hair day.

There is cake in the kitchen, you're thinking about going and having some – even though you know you are not really hungry.

If you could be in charge of how you are feeling it would be easier to eat better. Those emotional food cravings would stop ruling you.

This section can help you take charge.

How you feel

. . . affects your body.

. . . affects your metabolism and your energy levels.

. . . affects what you eat.

. . . affects how much exercise you will do.

When you are trying to lose weight, stress is the enemy working against you.

Learning how you can make yourself feel calmer and happier is essential for long-term weight loss.

Would you say that to a friend?

Notice what you say to yourself during the day.

You are probably saying horrible things.

Start to break the habit of being mean to yourself.

Break the habit of making yourself feel bad.

Negative thoughts drain your emotional and physical energy.

If you feel sad, anxious, alone, or incapable, you are more likely to turn to comfort food.

Think about something that you like about yourself.

Interrupt those bad thoughts.

Stress

The only explanation that your body has for stress is FAMINE.

As human beings we haven't evolved that far from our hunter-gatherer ancestors. Our bodies still think that the root cause of all stress is famine.

So when you are stressed your body will slow your metabolism down to save on food, thinking . . .

'Famine is coming – better stock up!'

Finding ways to reduce your stress levels will help keep your metabolism working at its optimum level – which will ultimately help you lose weight.

Try introducing a few minutes of a calming exercise like mindfulness (see pages 52–3) into your day.

What is mindfulness?

Mindfulness is a way of being present in the moment.

Being present in the moment means not trying to change anything; it means simply being aware.

Many of us are so busy – always thinking about what happened yesterday, and what we need to accomplish tomorrow – that we forget about the moment that we're in. We forget about now.

Being aware of *now* is about being present in a non-judgmental way.

It's a simple practice that can have big effects.

Brain time

Practise mindfulness

When you practise mindfulness – even for just a few minutes a day – you are allowing your head some recovery time. It gives your busy brain the chance to adjust and rebalance.

This will help you become free of the comfort foods you rely on to numb and soothe anxious thoughts.

Quieting your mind also allows it to reconnect with your body.

MINDFULNESS

Just five minutes of mindfulness a day will calm mind and body, reduce stress and make you feel happier. When your mind and body are more at peace you will feel better and eat better.

- **Sit or lie down. Close your eyes. Scan through your body with your mind, slowly starting from the top of your head just become aware of each part of your body, taking the time to notice how you are feeling physically. What parts are comfortable or uncomfortable? Now, in a non-judgemental way, notice how you are feeling emotionally. Are you grumpy, calm, stressed, happy, sad?**

- **Once you have done this start to focus on your breathing. Inhale and exhale deeply, in and out of your nose, as if you could breathe into the depths of your stomach.**

- After focusing on your breathing for a minute or two, take a deep breath in and as you exhale imagine counting the number one, in your mind. You may see the number in your mind's eye, or imagine that you can hear it. With your next out breath count the number two. Continue counting with each exhale up to ten, and then start again with one.

- As you count, keep your eyes closed and remain comfortably seated or lying down.

- Repeat counting from one to ten for five or ten minutes.

- As you do this you may find your mind drifting away. If you realise this is happening, just gently pull your mind back to counting and focusing on your breathing. This will become easier with practice.

BELIEFS ARE VERY POWERFUL

What do you believe?

- I have always failed at diets.

- I am always going to be big.

- I have a slow metabolism.

- It is hard to lose weight at my age.

- I have no will power.

- I just can't lose weight.

What is your strongest negative belief about your body and your weight?

Your mind works very hard to make your beliefs come true.

Think about the power that this belief has over you.

TAPPING OUT NEGATIVE BELIEFS

This will help your mind break down the negative beliefs that you no longer need.

Focus on one specific negative belief. Follow the tapping map (see pages 9–11), and repeat each statement out loud as you tap.

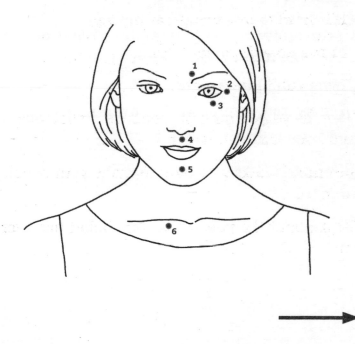

- **Even though I have this belief I am OK.**

- **Even though I believe that this is true I am OK.**

- **I know that this belief began for a reason, it is in the past now, I can move on.**

- **I can allow myself to imagine what it would be like to let this belief go.**

- **I can allow myself to imagine what it would feel like if this belief weren't true.**

- **This makes me feel _____ (energised, free, powerful, unburdened).**

MOOD BOOSTER

Remember: when you feel better, you eat better and you exercise more.

This is an easy mood booster to use when you feel a bit low.

- **Stand up.**

- **Breathe deeply.**

- **Look up, towards the sky.**

- **Stretch your hands up above your head, spreading your fingers apart.**

- **Smile (even if you don't feel like it).**

- **Smile (go on, show those teeth!).**

- **Smile at the world.**

- **As you exhale, gently lower your hands and shake them out.**

Being able to change
your mood is very
important.

Recognise that you are in
charge of your mood.

Your mood can determine your
metabolism.

Your mood affects
what you eat.

How does your mood affect your metabolism?

When you are in a **good mood** your serotonin levels are likely to be high (see page 39).

Not only do higher levels of serotonin benefit your overall happiness, they also suppress your appetite, causing you to eat small regular meals.

This type of eating boosts your metabolism.

When you are in a **bad mood**, it is likely that your serotonin levels are lower.

This will probably cause you to crave refined carbohydrates as they provide a short-term serotonin boost.

You will probably eat a large meal – and then nothing.

After several hours, your metabolism will slow down, as there is no food to process. As a result, you will also start to feel tired.

You will exercise less, which will, in turn, contribute to your metabolic slow down.

GROUNDING AND BREATHING

This quick exercise will help when you are feeling anxious or stressed. When your thoughts seem to be spinning around, you can use this technique to provide instant, on-the-spot calming.

- **Stand up and notice the weight of your feet on the ground. Make sure your knees are loose – not locked.**

- **Imagine that your feet are really planted into the ground, like the roots of a tall, strong oak tree.**

- **Now, allow your shoulders to relax gently away from your ears.**

- **Place one hand on your belly, and breathe deeply into the depths of your stomach. Imagine that this point, a couple of inches below your navel, is the very core of you.**

- **This is your navel centre or chakra, a centre of emotional well-being and the spot where much of the body's good energy or ch'i is stored.**

- **Stay in this position for a few breaths.**

This exercise is good for instant calming of mind and body.

Your unconscious mind is always working to make you happy

But sometimes, it gets it wrong.

For example, your unconscious mind wants you to feel happy and it knows that chocolate can do this. So it makes you crave chocolate when you are feeling down. What it doesn't know is that this is just a short-term fix. Relying on chocolate when you're down will, in reality, only make you gain weight – and, ultimately, this will make you unhappier.

Your mind needs to be re-educated – it needs to learn new ways of making you feel better.

Being aware of how your deeper mind is working against you means that you are already starting to make changes.

Stop pretending that your body isn't there

It is – and it's time you took some notice of it.

Are you drawing an invisible line at your neck – and ignoring what's below it?

You are not wearing an Elizabethan collar! Look down – your body is waiting.

Pay attention to it!

If you want to make changes to how your body looks you are going to have to start acknowledging that it is there.

How are you? (Yes, YOU)

Tune into your body. Reconnect with your body.

Do something nice for it,
>take a bubble bath,
>>lather on some lovely skin cream,
>>>>get a pedicure,
>>>>care for yourself.

When you care for your body you are more likely to take care of what you put *into* your body.

Love your body

'The curious paradox is that when I accept myself just as I am, then I can change.'
Carl Rogers, psychologist

If you hate your body and tell it so constantly, then it won't want to work with you to lose weight. Not to mention that you will be exhausted from this constant battle with yourself.

Showing love and acceptance to your body has energising effects. It enables it to work with you to create a slimmer, happier you.

LOVING YOUR BODY

- Close your eyes.

- With your fingertips gently tap the points on the inside edge of your eyebrows, then the outside edge of your eyebrows and, finally, tap below your eyes. Tap about eight times on each point (see diagram on page 11).

- As you do this, take deep breaths and think about your body – the amazing things it has allowed you to do, the places it has taken you, the people you have met.

- Keeping your eyes closed, place your right hand on your heart and your left hand on your stomach, below your belly button. Think appreciative, kind and loving thoughts towards your body.

- **As you breathe deeply, imagine the air from your inhale flowing from your heart down into your belly, and back again as you exhale.**

This is a yoga position, which links the heart and navel chakras. The navel chakra boosts feelings of confidence and self-esteem, while the heart chakra feels love and kindness. Encouraging these wonderful positive feelings within you will help you to love and care for your beautiful body.

MORNING WELLBEING BOOST

Get in the habit of doing this exercise in the shower every morning. It will give you a quick and easy energy boost, and will start you on the right path for the day ahead.

Using both of your hands, lightly tap each point for about 30 seconds with your fingertips.

- **Just below the points on your collarbone (1 and 2).**

- **Along the centre of your sternum (3).**

- **At the bottom of your ribs, in line with the nipples (4 and 5).**

- **Finally tap all over the top of your head like rain drops.**

- **Shake out your hands.**

These are strong acupressure points that will boost your wellbeing.

An adaptation of Donna Eden's Triple Thump from *Energy Medicine for Women*, Piatkus, 2009.

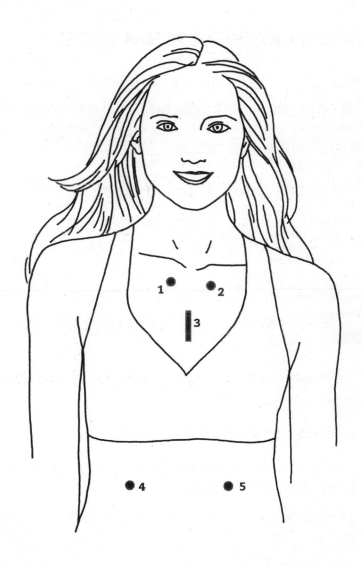

How do you want to look?

What does reaching your goal look like?

Toned Slim Healthy Gorgeous Fit Strong

Now, be honest: when you see others who are already at this weight how do you describe them?

Small Scrawny Ditzy Haggard Pathetic

Your mind will not let you achieve something you feel is negative.

If you are thinking negative thoughts towards slimmer people, start changing the message.

Turn it into something that your mind will want to achieve.

Are you the fairest of them all?

What happens when you look in the mirror?

Do you focus on the parts of your body that you hate?

What terrible thoughts are you thinking towards your body?

You need to get your body on your side. Look in the mirror and apologise to your body.

Yes, this is going to feel silly – but you really need to get your body working for you! Now say something nice to your body.

Look in the mirror and focus on a part of your body that you like. Perhaps it's your lovely hair, your beautiful eyes or your slim ankles. Recognise the good that already exists in your figure.

You are the fairest of them all.

When you are being kinder to your body, you will automatically take more care with what you put into it.

TAPPING AWAY THE POWER OF THE MIRROR

This exercise will help you to feel more confident in your appearance. For each statement, do one full circuit of the tapping map (see pages 9–11). Repeat each affirmation out loud as you tap.

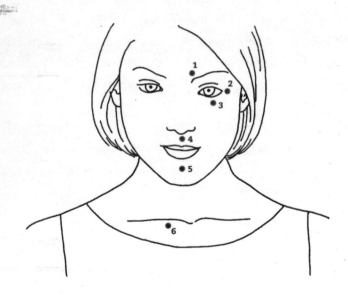

- I accept myself and how I look.

- I can allow myself to say nice things about how I look.

- I can look in the mirror and focus on the things I like about myself.

- I can allow myself to accept compliments.

- I can choose to stop making myself feel bad.

- I have the power to make myself feel good.

HOW DO I LOOK?

Close your eyes and imagine that you are standing naked in front of a full-length mirror.

When you hear that inner voice making those negative comments:

- **Repeat the comments out loud in a silly voice like Donald Duck.**

- **Answer the comments back – be strong, be confident.**

- **Now start to repeat the opposite comment to yourself – make that negative a positive!**

Example: 'You have fat legs – you look awful in trousers.'

Now becomes: 'I look great in trousers, my legs are becoming slimmer everyday.'

Begin to take more notice of that inner voice – it is chipping away at your self-esteem. When you learn to recognise it, you will take away its power over you.

WHO APPRECIATES YOU?

This exercise will help you to feel compassionate towards yourself.

- **Think about someone in your life who appreciates you just as you are.**

- **Close your eyes for a few moments and imagine they are standing in front of you, smiling and telling you that you are wonderful.**

- **Let yourself accept those positive thoughts – soak up the warmth of them, and keep that positive glow with you all day.**

Feel that love and appreciation for who you are.

The brain in your stomach

You have neurons in your stomach – this is why you can literally feel emotions in your gut.

So negative feelings – like anxiety, dread, sadness – register in the pit of your stomach.

Eating is a way that we try to push down and cover up these negative emotions.

Even though it can be scary sometimes, it is OK to face these negative thoughts and work through them.

When you deal with them you can begin to let them go.

You can be free of these negative emotions, which are causing you to eat much more than you need.

It might be that you need some positive emotional input.

The first step to being kind to your heart and mind is to look after your body. Become aware of just how important you are.

In order to gain control you must take responsibility for yourself.

It is not your mother's fault you are overweight.

It is not your partner's fault you are overweight.

It is not your job's fault you are overweight.

It is not your child's fault you are overweight.

It is not the dog's fault that you are overweight.

It is your fault.

This means you have the **power** to do something about it.

Because if it's not your fault, you are powerless, and that isn't something you want to be. When you take responsibility for yourself, your body and your emotions, you have the ability to change them.

You have power and control over your life.

In order to have
control of your life,
your body, your weight,
you must take responsibility
for yourself.

Only then can you make
changes.

When you are responsible you are in control.

Control

Are you willing to give control of your life over to others?

This can lead to depression and illness.

When you take back control you are letting go of the blame that you have put on others for all the things that have happened to you.

When you take control you have the power to change.

This can feel scary – but it can also feel energising, fantastic and wonderful.

Start taking control

By making a decision, you will feel empowered.

Start making decisions daily. Begin with small things and build up.

Say *no* to the things you don't want to do and *yes* to more of the things that you do want to do.

BREATHING FOR CALM

This yoga exercise quickly calms your mind and can help restore balance to your busy life.

It will relax you and reduce stress, which enables you to avoid comfort eating, and instead eat for health.

- **Stand or sit comfortably.**

- **Inhale through your nostrils and exhale slowly through your mouth.**

- **Exaggerate your breathing as you exhale making a 'haaaaaa' sound. Feel this sound reverberate at the back of your throat.**

- **Repeat several times.**

- **As you are exhaling just notice yourself letting go of heavy stresses and worries, letting your shoulders drop a little each time and as you inhale, imagine breathing in a light, calm feeling.**

Stress changes your brain chemistry

- When all else in life is chaos the one thing you have control over is what you are going to put into your body.

- This is another reason why you can find yourself turning to food for comfort.

- It is this control aspect of food that can also lead to eating disorders.

- Remember that you are the boss of what you eat.

- You need to teach your mind and body that there are better ways to lower stress.

The chemicals at work in your body – cortisol

When your body is under stress it releases extra amounts of a hormone called cortisol.

This is the same hormone that prepares your body for 'fight or flight'.

Evolutionarily speaking, this is a very important response. But when your body experiences long-term exposure to high levels of cortisol there are negative effects:

- Higher blood pressure
- Decrease in muscle tissue
- Lowered immunity
- Decrease in bone density
- Altered blood sugar levels
- Detrimental impact on fertility
- Reduction in serotonin levels.

Your brain under stress

If you want to lose weight and keep it off, you'll need to learn how to reduce your stress levels.

- Stress increases the levels of cortisol in the brain.

- This can cause you to crave comfort foods.

- Comfort foods will seem to temporarily dull the stress for a short time.

- But these same comfort foods also lead to an over-production of insulin – and, as a result, your blood sugar levels will soon begin to plunge.

- You will feel tired, irritable and crave more comfort food.

- You will gain weight.

Remember: Practising mindfulness can help to dramatically reduce your stress levels.

SECTION 4

Understanding Your Food Rules

You live your life by a series of rules or habits. You brush your teeth in the morning. You call your mother on Thursdays. Once a month you have a girls' night out.

You also have food rules – patterns and habits that your mind has programmed in and that you now perform automatically.

When I start to talk about this on my weight loss course I see a look of realisation spreading around the room as people begin to think about the things that they do automatically week after week. In some cases it has been always getting chocolate at a petrol station, or finishing the children's toast every morning.

Learning about your own food rules is a crucial component of changing the way you look, as these are the habits that may be keeping you stuck where you are.

As you begin to make changes you may find yourself craving certain foods. For example, you might always have crisps while watching TV on a Friday night. You try and stop eating crisps and find you are left with a craving for them. Your mind expects this food, it wants this food, the craving gets stronger and stronger. Part of this section deals with food cravings which will help you change your food rules.

What are your food rules?

- I always have cereal and toast in the morning.

- I always have a curry on a Friday night.

- I always have a biscuit with a cup of tea.

- I always get popcorn when I see a film.

- I always eat everything on my plate.

Are your food rules ruling you?

These are the habits that are keeping you at your current weight.

BREAK YOUR FOOD RULES

Make a list of your current food rules.

Now make a separate list of some new alternatives that you would be happier with.

I always have a
biscuit with a cup
of tea I choose to have
a piece of fruit
with my tea.

Be aware of these old rules, and begin to implement the new ones.

The first time you make a change it may feel difficult, but each time after this it will become easier and easier.

Beware the clean plate club.

No lives were ever saved by someone clearing all the food off their plate.

When you are no longer hungry . . .

STOP EATING.

TAPPING INTO YOUR ABILITY
TO CREATE BETTER FOOD RULES

This exercise will help you to break free of your
negative patterns.

Follow the points on the tapping map (see pages
9–11) and do one round for each affirmation.
Repeat each statement out loud as you tap.

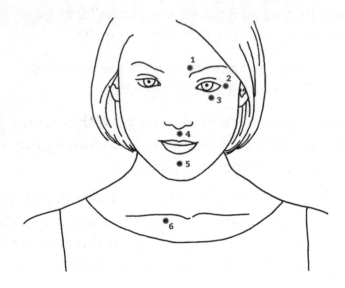

- Even though I don't think I can change my food rules, I am OK.

- Even though it feels hard to change, I accept myself.

- (Rubbing the Sore Spot (see page 130)) I have always done this and it feels as if I always will.

- (Returning to the other points on the tapping map) Even though I can't imagine doing something different, I am OK.

- Even though this won't help me to change my food rules, I accept myself.

- Even though it's hard to let go of this excess weight that's stopping me from having the life I want, I accept myself.

When it feels as though part of you wants to keep a certain habit or belief while another part of you wants to change, rubbing the Sore Spot helps to overcome a resistance to change.

A MOMENT OF CALM

Sometimes there just aren't enough hours in the day for quality 'me time'. This two-minute exercise will give your mind and body a quick boost, calming you and allowing you to put life into perspective. Letting your mind have this break will give it the strength it needs to consciously recognise and change your food rules.

- **Place your right hand on your heart.**

- **Place your left hand on your stomach, just below your belly button.**

- **Close your eyes and breathe deeply through your nose.**

- **Gently drop your shoulders away from your ears.**

- **Send yourself a compliment.**

    'I am a good friend'   'I am a caring mother'
        'I work hard'   'I am an honest person'

- **Bask in this compliment for a few moments before opening your eyes and going on with your day.**

FOOD CRAVING BREAK

Do you find yourself craving a specific food, at a specific time, locked into a food rule?

Try doing the exercise below to break down the strength of that craving:

- **Place your right hand on the centre of your chest.**

- **Rub the skin between the bones of the fourth and fifth fingers of your right hand with the fingers of your left hand, the Gamut point.**

- **As you rub this point focus your mind on the food that you have been craving.**

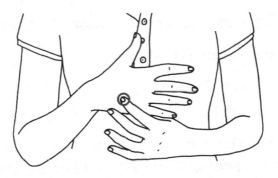

Stimulating these acupressure points helps to calm the mind and reduce the craving.

Are you having constant food cravings?

Have you been ignoring physical hunger? Skipping meals?

If so, your body will start craving foods that will give it a fast sugar boost.

Remember, if you eat refined sugars and carbohydrates your blood sugar will only temporarily lift before crashing – leaving you feeling tired, low, irritable and craving more food.

As a result, you will eat more than you need – and, inevitably, you will gain weight.

You have a choice.

Change your routine.

Interrupt the cycle.

Have a new plan.

TAPPING ON CRAVINGS – BREAK DOWN THOSE ATTACHMENTS

This tapping exercise helps you to separate emotions from food and break down the links to the food you are craving. It is these links that make your mind believe that this food is going to help you feel better, when in fact it is now doing just the opposite.

Follow the points on the tapping map (see pages 9–11) and do one round for each statement. Repeat each statement out loud as you tap, filling in the blank with the food you are craving.

⟶

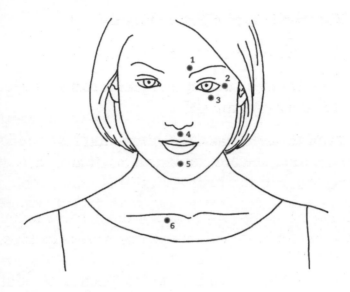

- **Even though I have a craving, I am OK.**

- **Even though I really want to eat _____, I am OK.**

- **Even though I don't want to give up this food, I accept myself.**

- **Even though I don't feel I can give up this craving, I am OK.**

- **This food helps me in some way.**

- **It makes me feel better.**

- **Even though I do not feel I have control over this craving, I am OK.**

- **Even though I can't imagine what I will do without this food, I accept myself and that feels good.**

Finish by using both hands to tap across the top of your head, as if your fingertips were raindrops.

QUICK CRAVING TAP

When you find yourself standing in the kitchen deciding whether or not you are going to give into a craving, this exercise will help you make a quick emotional shift.

Begin tapping at your temple, following the skin behind the ears and down the sides of your neck, ending as you reach the tops of your shoulders.

Left-hand side

As you tap repeat this phrase five times:

I no longer like the taste of _____ .

Right-hand side

As you tap repeat this phrase five times:

I love being free from craving _____ .

Developed by George Goodheart, the founder of applied kinesiology and Donna Eden in *Energy Medicine for Women*, Piatkus, 2009.

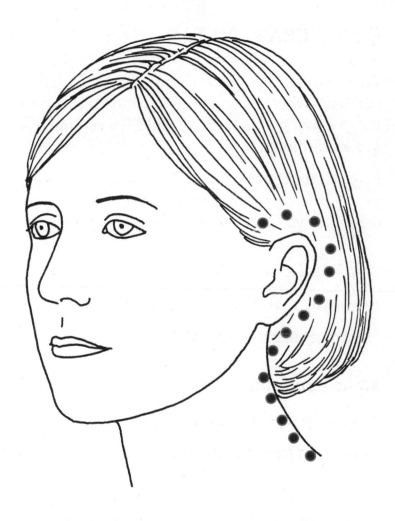

SECTION 5

Overcoming Emotional Eating

You fall over when you are little and Mum gives you a biscuit. Gran gets you a special cake as a treat whenever you visit her. When you have had a stressful day chocolate seems to help.

We all do it, we all use food to make us feel better.

Or at least that is what we think it's doing.

But it gets to a point when eating this way is no longer making you feel better, but there doesn't seem to be a way to change.

I have used the techniques in this section to help many people break free from a lifetime of emotional eating. Enabling them to feel happier, freer and slimmer.

'There aren't enough cookies in the world to make you feel loved and whole'

Michael Neill, bestselling author and life coach
www.supercoach.com

Food cravings = emotional hunger

TURNING OFF EMOTIONAL HUNGER

This exercise will activate the energy in your stomach and allow your mind to be aware of how it is feeling, helping you to distinguish between physical and emotional hunger.

- **Stand comfortably with your arms by your sides.**

- **Slowly lift your arms. When they are above your head reach back as far as is comfortable. Feel the stretch in your stomach before returning to a neutral, upright position.**

- **Slowly lower your arms and repeat three times.**

Take care with this exercise if you have back problems.

TAPPING OUT EMOTIONAL EATING

Begin tapping at your temple, following the skin behind the ears and down the sides of your neck, ending as you reach the tops of your shoulders.

Left-hand side

As you tap repeat this phrase five times:

Negative feelings no longer cause me to overeat.

Right-hand side

As you tap repeat this phrase five times:

I eat for health and for a slim body.

Developed by George Goodheart, the founder of applied kinesiology and Donna Eden in *Energy Medicine for Women*.

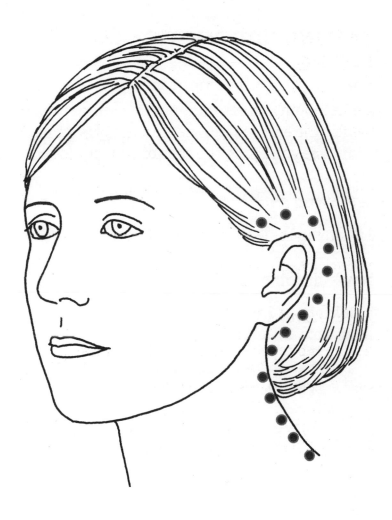

EXTEND YOUR VIEW

Imagine you are looking at some very tempting, highly fattening food.

You want it, you deserve it, you need a bit – after all it's been a hard week.

It's really easy to talk yourself into eating it.

But you are only thinking about the next 30 seconds of your life.

Now – imagine your perspective is changing.

Think about how you'll feel 30 minutes from now. Now envision yourself in 30 days.

What do you want to be doing then? What do you want to be wearing?

Think about how this type of food will stop you from achieving your goal. Now, the food becomes less appealing, even disgusting.

You see it for what it really is: momentary pleasure but long-term sabotage, which will only lead to guilt and a sense of failure.

How different does that food look when you see the real outcome?

You can choose not to eat it, and feel satisfied as a result.

You can choose.

WHEN DO YOU OVEREAT?

Make a list of the times, situations or places where you regularly overeat.

It could be when you get home at the end of the day – going straight to the kitchen and filling up with junk food.

Now come up with a new plan – write down something else that you could do in each scenario, something that would make you feel better about yourself.

You might decide to make a cup of tea when you come in and to run a bubble bath to relax in.

It's easier to make a plan when you are not in the moment.

Now when that situation next arises you can choose to do something else that will make you feel good. Your mind will already have an alternative route that it can choose to follow.

CRAVING COMFORT FOOD?

If you are feeling low and craving comfort food, try rubbing the area of skin just below the nail on the little finger of your left hand. Gently rub from the inside of the nail towards the ring finger to the outside edge of the nail.

Repeat this action for a minute.

This is a strong acupressure point and can help to ease low moods.

The diet tightrope

As you learn new techniques to help you lose weight and to make changes in your life that will keep the weight off for good, you are also letting go of that stressful diet tightrope you used to try and balance on.

You are now walking along a new path, and it's one that allows you to make some mistakes.

When you make a mistake now – and you will because you are only human – it no longer means falling off that tightrope. Instead, you are just wandering from side-to-side, on that new wider path, before you straighten out again.

What does this mean?

It means that when you have some chocolate now, you have a little bit. You don't feel that huge sense of failure and then just succumb to it by eating the entire bar. Now, you enjoy a small piece and put the rest away.

TAPPING OUT YOUR ATTACHMENT TO COMFORT FOODS

This exercise will help you to break out of a cycle of emotional eating.

Follow the points on the tapping map (see pages 9–11) and do one round for each statement. Repeat each affirmation out loud as you tap.

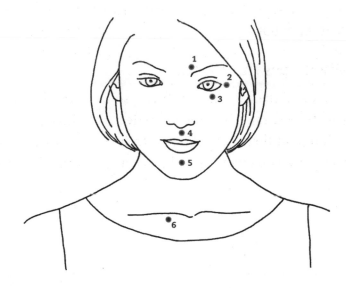

- Even though I comfort eat, I accept myself.

- Even though I have done this for so long, I am OK.

- Even though I am worried that I won't be able to stop comfort eating, I am OK.

- It's scary to imagine life without comfort eating.

- I can't imagine choosing to do something else.

- It could feel good to let this comfort eating go.

- I can allow myself to be free of comfort eating, it was an old habit that I no longer need.

Some days you will fail.

Expect it.
Accept it.
You are only human.
It is OK.

Forgive yourself.

CRAVING BLASTER

Use this exercise when you just can't seem to break free from a craving – and it's driving you nuts!

- **Stand up.**

- **Put your arms out in front of you, palms up, bend your elbows and make your hands into fists.**

- **Think about the craving you want to let go of.**

- **Take in a deep breath and as you do swing your arms up behind you and above your head.**

- **As you loudly exhale swing your arms down in front of you, opening up your hands with your palms facing upwards.**

- **Repeat three times.**

- **End by placing one hand on your heart and the other on your belly. Close your eyes and take three deep breaths, inhaling and exhaling through your nose.**

- **You will find yourself feeling happier, lighter and freer.**

Derived from Donna Eden's Blow-out technique in *Energy Medicine for Women*.

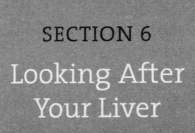

SECTION 6

Looking After
Your Liver

Your liver is your body's personal washing machine.

The liver's job is to cleanse toxins from the body.

But the liver has to prioritise the toxins it deals with.

If there is alcohol in the body, the liver targets that first.

When your liver is busy absorbing alcohol it cannot process the excess fat that you have been trying so hard to get rid of.

As a result you don't lose any weight.

It's just a drink...

When alcohol comes into the body the liver breaks it down.

Alcohol intake reduces the liver's ability to remove fat from your blood, and also causes it to increase its production of triglycerides.

Triglycerides contain fat.

An excess of triglycerides can be stored as fat in the liver. This could result in fatty liver disease.

Fatty deposits on your liver also reduce its efficiency in removing toxins from your body.

Excessive amounts of triglycerides in the body can also increase the risk of strokes and heart attacks.

When your body is busy processing alcohol it's not processing food or fat.

The result?
You don't lose any weight.

Alcohol wears your body out and keeps you out of the clothes you want to wear.

Alcohol raises the levels of cortisol – the stress hormone – in your body.

Excessive levels of cortisol can lead to sleep problems and a decrease in muscle mass.

In turn, poor sleep causes further hormone imbalances, which can increase your appetite and desire for comfort foods.

Alcohol can cause you to lose muscle mass and to eat more food.

A fatty belly can mean a fatty liver

Excess body fat is often indicative of an overworked liver.

Things that tire out a liver:

Alcohol   Sugar   Caffeine

Processed foods   Refined carbohydrates

Fatty foods

Go on – give your liver a break.

When you drink alcohol, your body relies on it for energy, instead of burning fat.

It will also make you search for food to nibble on.

Drink less and you will burn more fat.

What is a glass of wine?

It's pasta in a glass!!!!

(Do you *really* want that Chardonnay now?)

SUPPORTING YOUR LIVER

Hold your right hand with your left hand. With a gentle, circular motion use the thumb of your left hand to massage the palm of your right hand.

Do this for two minutes.

Repeat twice daily.

This is a reflexology technique that can help support your liver.

GET THAT LIVER ENERGY MOVING

Place your finger on the skin between your big toe and the second toe.

Pressing gently, move your finger up towards your ankle. You will feel a small dip about 3 cm up your foot.

Gently press this point for a minute to help promote the liver.

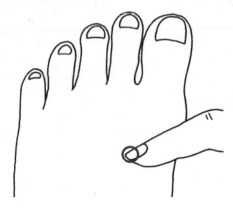

This is a strong acupressure point, Liv-3, that when activated, helps rebalance the liver.

Whenever possible eat foods in their natural state.

An apple...

Not apple pie!

This will put less stress on your liver and give you more energy.

As you eat healthier
and exercise more frequently
your body will clear out toxins.

You will find that you have more
energy.

You will look younger and more
vibrant.

You will feel better –
emotionally and
physically.

QUICK TOXIN RELEASE EXERCISE

There is a spot in the dip below your collarbone and next to your shoulder which can feel slightly sensitive when touched, also known as the Sore Spot.

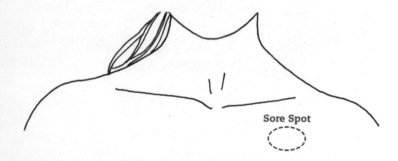

Rubbing this spot in a circular motion on each side of your body for a minute activates an acupressure meridian that will help to release lymphatic congestion, helping to clear out waste from your body.

Fewer Toxins = More Energy

SECTION 7

Self-Hypnosis: Using the Power of Your Mind

If this section makes you nervous, relax!

This is not something you have to learn.

You are actually already an expert at self-hypnosis.

Your mind uses automatic trances – which is another term for self-hypnosis – to lock you into repeating certain behaviour.

When you're in this state, your conscious mind gets a break.

More often than not, these trances are one of the many ways that our brains look after us – enabling us to function while simultaneously giving us a rest. Your thoughts can wander while you drive for miles on the same road, and you automatically brush your teeth every morning, sometimes when you're only barely awake.

But automatic trances can also cause problems. They can keep you stuck in negative patterns, without you even realising what's happening.

Your automatic food trances

Have you ever found yourself looking at an empty packet of food that you ate without tasting, without even noticing?

You were in a trance.

You mind has trances that it will lock you into, causing you to repeat behaviour.

Shopping in the supermarket and automatically picking up the same brands of toilet paper or jam, zoning out while watching TV...

...or eating the contents of the fridge when you're stressed.

After eating the food you find yourself 'waking up' and becoming aware of what you have done. This happens to smokers and it is just as much of a problem for binge eaters.

Break your trance

In order to regain control you need to break this trance.
Do something that your mind doesn't expect.

Wake your mind up!

Just before your deeper mind takes over there is a moment when you can break out of your trance. A moment just before you stuff your face with food you don't need.

Try:

Star jumps   **Stamping your feet**
Clapping your hands   **Shouting at yourself**

The first time you break the trance it will feel difficult, but each subsequent time you break the trance you are weakening the power it has over you.

Positive trances

It is possible to use the power of a trance to help you achieve your weight loss goal.

You can harness the power of your mind and get it to work for you. This is a positive trance, and a form of self-hypnosis.

How does this work?

When your mind imagines something over and over again it begins to believe that it has really happened.

We have all had the experience of waking up from a dream and not knowing whether it was real or not. So if your mind has imagined over and over again that you are slim and healthy – then it will look for ways of making it a reality.

By using mindfulness you have already practised putting yourself into a wonderfully calming trance-type state. This is the beginning of self-hypnosis.

IMAGINING YOUR GOAL

Creating your goal as a strong force in your mind is extremely powerful. It will function like a huge magnet in your future, pulling you towards it – giving you the confidence and determination to achieve your target weight.

Read through the rest of the page and then allow your imagination to create a powerful vision of how it will feel to achieve a slimmer, healthier body.

Use the mindfulness technique on pages 52–3 to help you relax.

Allow your mind to quiet down as you begin to focus on your breathing.

While in this relaxed state simply allow yourself to imagine that you have achieved your goal.

You are wearing the clothes you want to wear. Notice how people are responding to this new, slimmer you – how wonderful it feels to go about your day in this slim, healthy body.

Imagine shopping for clothes and choosing to try something on in exactly the right size for this slimmer you. Feel the sensation of the clothes as you put them on – feel how they skim over your body and fit you wonderfully.

Perhaps you catch sight of yourself in the mirror, and notice just how good you look.

Enjoy this feeling. Now notice the date on the calendar – this is the date you are going to achieve your goal by.

You find yourself smiling because you know that this is going to happen.

Now open your eyes.

REHEARSAL OF AN EVENING OUT

When you are at home you can be in control of what you are eating. But when you go out for dinner, it can feel as if you have been thrown into the deep water and don't know how to swim. You may feel waves of anxiety hitting you as you see all that is on offer before you.

First, use the technique of mindfulness to quiet your thoughts (see pages 52–3).

Once you feel calm and inwardly focused allow yourself to imagine that you are getting ready to go out. You can visualise the evening unfolding as if you were watching it on film.

You can imagine arriving at the restaurant where you will be eating. See yourself sitting down at the table. You are composed and confident.

Notice how you choose food and drinks that will help you achieve your goal of a slimmer you.

You feel in control. It seems so easy to choose healthy food.

Notice also how you stop eating when you are no longer hungry – putting your knife and fork down and perhaps allowing food to be left on your plate.

At the end of the meal you feel happy, relaxed and satisfied.

Open your eyes.

Repeat this exercise several times before going out for a meal.

PREPARING FOR A STRESSFUL SITUATION

Sometimes you know that an upcoming event is going to cause you stress. It might be the situation itself – perhaps a formal work event, or a presentation – or, perhaps, it's the people who will surround you and the prospect of having to spend time with someone you don't really get along with.

Even if you can't control the event that causes the stress, using self-hypnosis, you *can* reduce the effect that it is going to have on you and your eating pattern. You can teach that deeper part of your mind how you want to behave.

Come to a calm and inwardly focused state, using mindfulness (see pages 52–3), and allow yourself to think about the situation.

Watch yourself as you go through the entire meeting – from your preparation for it until you come home.

As you do this, allow the tranquillity that you are experiencing in this state of mindfulness to change how you imagine yourself feeling and behaving during the event.

Notice if you respond differently to people.

Run through the event in your mind several times, allowing for a variety of potentially stressful scenarios. Picture yourself responding with control, ease and grace.

Notice how calmly you are able to cope.

Open your eyes.

Each time you carry this exercise out you might find that you respond in better, calmer ways to the situation. And when it comes to the actual day, you will find yourself feeling collected, relaxed and able to cope well.

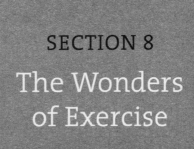

SECTION 8

The Wonders
of Exercise

Many of my overweight clients have a gym membership and come into their first session saying that they hate the gym but they are going to start going regularly after seeing me.

I ask, 'Why?'

If you hate the gym please stop paying the fees!

There are so many other types of exercise you could be doing – you just need to find the one that you enjoy. Otherwise you are not going to keep doing it.

Walking, swimming, running, dancing, cycling, yoga, tennis, sailing, rowing, judo, horse-riding . . .

Exercise:

Burns calories – when you exercise you are burning extra calories, which will help you reach your goal.

Boosts metabolism – this means you will continue burning extra calories even when you have finished exercising.

Makes your brain happy – as you exercise you release endorphins, which make you feel good.

Gets you into shape – exercise can help prevent heart disease and strokes, lower blood pressure, improve bone density and reduce the risk of diabetes.

Does this sound familiar?

My metabolism is slowing down.

I'm getting older.

I can't lose weight.

Rubbish!

In reality you are probably doing less load bearing exercise, and as a result, you have much less muscle mass – this is what is causing your metabolism to slow down.

The best way to speed up your metabolism?

Get moving!

Your metabolism:

- Is not fixed.
- It can change with what you eat and with exercise.

When your diet is restrictive and you skip meals your body thinks that it is in a time of famine – and this makes your metabolism slow down, in order to conserve energy.

Keep dieting and you will keep gaining weight.

Stop starving your body.

Eat to lose weight!

Water Water Water

If you are dehydrated your body will feel tired.

Your metabolism will slow down.

You will have a false sensation of hunger.

Remember to keep hydrated when you are exercising.

Before you reach for that snack, drink a glass of water!

Exercising can double your metabolic rate.

But you must be exercising enough to get sweaty and out of breath!

GET THAT STUCK ENERGY MOVING!

Your brain is a centre of energy, and, sometimes, it needs a boost.

If you are feeling sluggish you need to get this energy moving.

Your head is covered in acupressure points which when massaged will invigorate your mind and body.

- **Sit somewhere comfortable.**

- **Become aware of your breathing as you inhale and exhale deeply and slowly. Imagine that you can follow the path of your breath as you do this.**

- **Begin massaging your forehead, cheeks and gently around the eyes.** (A)

- **Now slowly and with a light pressure begin to massage your scalp with your fingertips, continuing down to the base of your neck.**
  (B, C, D)

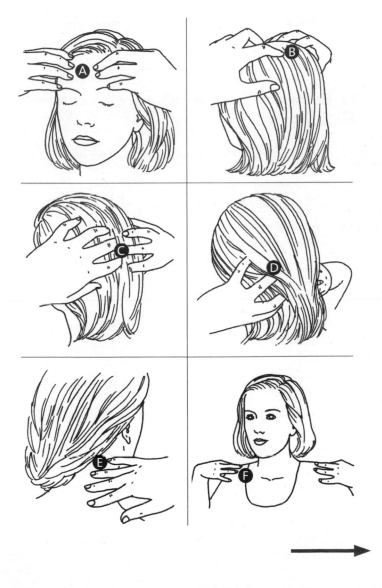

- **Finally run your fingers down your neck to your shoulders and relax your hands.** (E, F)

- **While breathing deeply, take a few moments to notice any changes in how you are now feeling.**

BOOSTING YOUR IMMUNE SYSTEM

When you are feeling stronger in mind and body you will have more energy for exercise.

This acupressure exercise can help to reinforce your immune system:

- **Place your fingers on the points that stick out on your collarbone.**

- **Just below these, on the top part of your chest, you will feel slight depressions.**

- **Firmly press these points as you breathe deeply for one minute.**

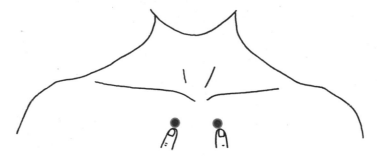

In acupressure, these are known as the K-27 points.

When you do something for six weeks it becomes a habit.

Do something for three months and it will become a way of life.

What does this mean for you?

At first it might be difficult to put in place that new way of eating or new exercise regime.

But persist – in just a few short weeks you will find it becomes easier and very soon it will become effortless – simply a part of your daily routine.

You will find yourself *automatically* eating better and exercising more.

Exercise releases
tension and stress.

Exercise also releases
endorphins – those wonderful
mood boosting chemicals.

So after a workout you feel
calmer and happier!

When you are happier you
eat healthier and eat less.

TAPPING INTO YOUR METABOLISM

This exercise will boost your metabolism and make you feel more energetic – ready to exercise!

Follow the points on the tapping map (see pages 9–11) and do one full circuit for each statement. Repeat each statement out loud as you tap.

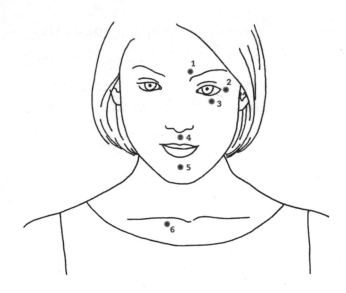

- Even though I feel my metabolism has been slow, I am OK.

- I can let go of whatever has been slowing down my metabolism.

- I can allow my metabolism to speed up.

- I can feel energy beginning to pump through my body; my body is burning more calories.

- My metabolism is now speeding up to the perfect rate for me.

Note: This exercise should be done in the morning. If carried out at night it may affect sleep.

TAPPING OUT NEGATIVE EXERCISE THOUGHTS

This exercise will help you break free of those old negative thoughts and feelings towards exercise. It will allow you to feel more positive towards exercise.

Follow the points on the tapping map (see pages 9–11) and do one full circuit for each statement. Repeat each statement out loud as you tap.

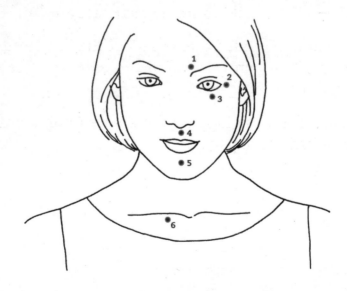

- **Even though I don't really feel like exercising, I am OK.**

- **Even though I don't want to go and exercise, I am OK.**

- **I am tired and I accept myself.**

- **Even though I haven't got the energy to exercise, I am OK.**

- **Even though I find exercising difficult, I accept myself.**

- **Even though it is scary to change, I am OK.**

As you finish this exercise repeat the last statement while gently rubbing the Sore Spot (see page 130).

Finally finish by tapping the Karate Chop point eight times (see page 11).

STILL FEELING NEGATIVE ABOUT EXERCISE?

Tapping will help you shift those negative emotions.

Begin tapping at your temple, following the skin behind the ears and down the sides of your neck, ending as you reach the tops of your shoulders.

Left-hand side

As you tap repeat this phrase five times:

I am no longer negative when I think about exercise.

Right-hand side

As you tap repeat this phrase five times:

I enjoy exercise. When I exercise I feel great.

Developed by George Goodheart, the founder of applied kinesiology and Donna Eden in *Energy Medicine for Women*.

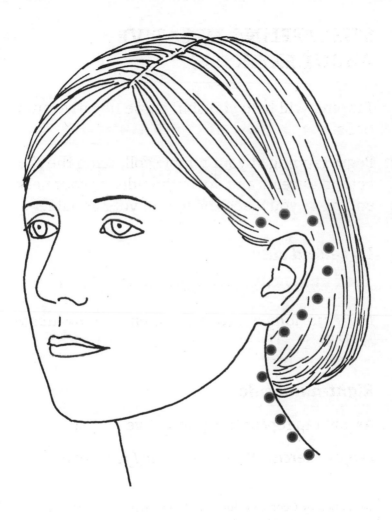

Walking

Sedentary people walk less than
5,000 steps a day.

Active people walk about
10,000 steps a day.

Get a pedometer!!!

It has been shown that wearing
a pedometer will help increase
the number of steps you take
each day.

Just a few extra steps a day could
make a huge difference to your
life and your health.

As discussed in 'How many steps a day are enough?: Preliminary
pedometer indices for public health' by C. Tudor-Locke and D. R.
Bassett in *Sports Medicine,* Vol. 34(1), 1–8, 2004.

WANT TO EXERCISE – BUT FEELING SLUGGISH? TRY THIS ENERGY TAP

This energy tap will give you a mental and physical boost, helping you to find the energy and motivation to exercise.

- **Start by breathing deeply in and out through your nose.**

- **Place your fingers on your forehead and gently massage the skin.** (A)

- **Continue to gently massage your temples.** (B) **Now use all ten fingers to tap across the top of your scalp, like raindrops.** (C)

- **Using your index fingers tap on the inside edge of your eyebrows eight times.** (D)

- **Repeat on the outside edge of your eyes and then under each eye.** (E)

⟶

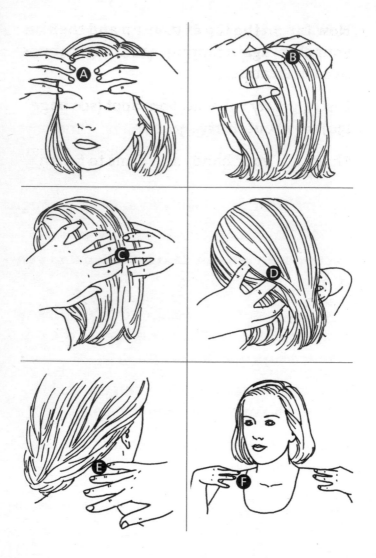

- Now tap on the top of your lip and then on your chin, again tapping about eight times in each location. (F)

- Lastly, gently rub your Sore Spot (see page 130) for about thirty seconds.

- Shake out your hands and arms to finish.

Remember that you will have slip-ups – You are not perfect. You are only human.

When you accept this you don't have to waste energy beating yourself up about mistakes. You don't have to give up on your plan for the day or week just because you were running late and had a muffin for breakfast – you can shrug it off and nudge yourself back onto your correct path.

Spending less energy worrying means you have more energy for exercise and making yourself healthier!

Oxygen Oxygen Oxygen

Boost Your Oxygen Levels and Boost Your Weight Loss.

Breathing seems like the most natural, effortless thing we do. But paying attention to how we breathe is very important.

- Breathing deeply can boost your metabolism and give you more energy for exercise.

- This means you will burn more calories!

- Each time you exhale you breathe out toxins.

- By breathing deeply you are stimulating your lymphatic system which helps to remove even more toxins from your body.

- Deep breathing provides the cells of your body with oxygen, especially your intestines, which promotes your body's ability to absorb nutrients.

Most of us take only shallow breaths. When you are shallow breathing only the top of your chest will move. But when you are breathing deeply, the top of your chest will be still and your stomach will move in and out.

→

To access your deep breathing, imagine that as you inhale, you are following the air as it travels down into your stomach and following the same breath out again as you exhale. Try to take ten deep breaths like this, three times a day for maximum benefit.

POWERFUL BREATHING

This exercise will greatly boost your oxygen levels.

- **Stand up.**

- **Make one hand into a fist and place it gently at the bottom of your ribs.**

- **Place your other hand on top of the fist and gently pull in.**

- **Inhale deeply through your nose, feeling the pressure of your breath against your hands. Relax your fist as you exhale through your mouth.**

- **Repeat ten times.**

- **You will feel a surge of energy in mind and body.**

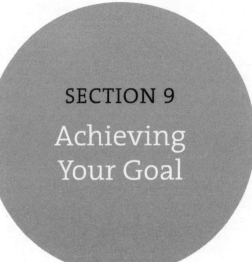

SECTION 9

Achieving
Your Goal

Your goal is to lose weight – to become that slim, healthy you that you have dreamt about for so long.

In order to achieve your goal it is important to stay focused on what you want, and to know where you are going.

It is also important to understand the blocks to weight loss that might be standing in your way. If you can begin to recognise these obstacles then you can consciously face them and overcome them.

I have worked with many people who have become aware of an issue that has been blocking their weight loss – it is almost as if a light has gone on inside their mind. Suddenly they see what has been going on and in that moment everything changes – and they start moving towards their goal.

Once you are consciously aware of what has been holding you back you can face it and make the changes you need to.

The pounds start to melt away because there is no longer a reason to keep them.

You goal becomes a reality.

How will you know when you have reached your goal?

Is it by the number on the scales?

How many miles you are able to run?

Fitting into a certain pair of jeans?

When do you want to achieve your goal?

In a month?   6 months?   12 months?

Take some time to think about this and set a realistic date.

If you don't know where you are going you are never going to get there.

WHAT IS STOPPING YOU?

What has been preventing you from losing that excess weight?

Imagine you have reached your goal: you are the size, weight and shape that you want to be.

Just close your eyes and experience this for a few minutes. Imagine being in that body. Take the time to be fully aware of how it would feel to be in this new body.

How does it *really* feel to be this size?

- **Are there any negative feelings about being this size?**

- **Is there anything you have promised yourself you will do when you are this slim?**

- **Anything you might be nervous about actually doing?**

- **Is there anyone in your life who is not happy about what you have achieved or about the way you look?**

Think about how you would deal with any negativity that arises once you have achieved your goal. If you are prepared for a negative reaction then it will not set you back. You will be able to deflect it and feel happy within yourself.

Promises

Take a few moments to think about the things you have promised yourself you will do when you are slim.

You might have vowed that you'll buy new clothes or finally try a new haircut.

Or you might have promised yourself that you will make a bigger change:

- Perhaps go back to college and enrol in the course you have always wanted to take.

- Get a new job – one that really challenges you or that you are more passionate about.

- Start dating again.

Sometimes we promise ourselves things that we really, truly want, but that also make us a bit nervous.

If you are aware that there is something you might be nervous of doing once you are slim, then you can take the steps now to begin to become more confident about whatever it is that you want to do. Take small steps to achieve your big goal – get a brochure for that college course, talk to a recruitment consultant about possible career moves, or ask a friend to set you up with one of their single friends.

Are you comfortable with change?

As you lose weight and move towards that new body shape, the shape you have always wanted, you are creating change.

These changes in yourself – how you feel and how you look – may also lead to changes in how you are perceived and treated by others.

Change can cause you to feel nervous and you may want to retreat back into the familiar.

This means gaining back the weight you have lost.

This may make you feel safe again – and it may have happened in the past without you even realising what was going on.

But now that you are becoming more aware of how your mind and body are connected, you are learning new ways of being which will enable you to cope with the anxieties that change awakens. You can embrace the new slimmer, healthier, happier you with confidence.

If you are not comfortable with the new you, no one else will be.

Becoming comfortable with the new you is very important.

You deserve to enjoy this new slimmer you.

Negative people

It's hard to imagine that there would be people in your life who might respond negatively to your weight loss.

But there might be.

Being aware of what is causing that negative emotion will help you to overcome it – and to feel confident about what you are achieving for yourself.

* Sometimes friends can feel threatened by the 'new you' and will want to push you back into that old shape so they feel comfortable in their life again.

* Partners can be jealous of the attention your new slimmer figure might attract. Or they may worry that you might leave them as your confidence grows.

* Family members – mothers, fathers, siblings – may also make negative comments about your new look. Your weight loss might be highlighting their own insecurities.

TAPPING OUT BLOCKS TO WEIGHT LOSS

This exercise will help you move forward to a slimmer you.

Follow the points on the tapping map (see pages 9–11) and do one full circuit for each statement. Repeat each statement out loud as you tap.

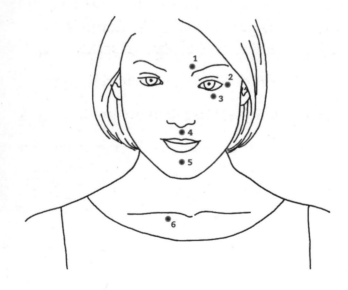

- Even though I am nervous about being slim, I am OK.

- There may be reasons why I haven't let myself be slim before but I can choose to let those go now.

- I can allow myself to move on.

- I am stronger now and I can enjoy being slimmer.

- I am not the person I was – I am more confident now and I accept myself.

- I can allow myself to be slim and happy.

- I can allow myself to reach my goal.

Set the date you will achieve your goal

Put the date you are going to achieve your goal into your calendar.

Think about the changes that are already starting to happen in your life that will allow you to easily achieve this goal.

You might need to add in the dates of some other things you are going to do during the same period of time that will keep you moving towards this ultimate objective.

As you approach this date keep checking on your progress. Continue making the changes you need to in order to achieve the results you want when you want them.

Smile – you can feel good about yourself.

You are changing, you are making this happen.

You are important.

You are important.

You are important.

Get it?

What if you are important?

Then it is important that you look after yourself.

It is important that you pay attention to how you are feeling.

If you are important then you give yourself time to exercise.

If you are important then every morsel that goes into your body matters.

**This is not a diet –
this is a change of lifestyle.**

You may slip off your path occasionally,
but when you do, remember it's OK – pick up
Diet Coach and there will be assistance and
encouragement waiting.

**You deserve to be happy and slim, and
you can be.**

'It's never too late to become what you might have been'

George Eliot

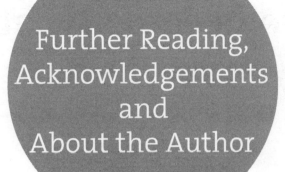

Further Reading,
Acknowledgements
and
About the Author

Further Reading

Jack Challem, *The Food Mood Solution*, John Wiley, 2007

Donna Eden, *Energy Medicine for Women*, Piatkus, 2009

Susan Jeffers, *Feel the Fear and Do It Anyway*, Vermilion, 2007

David A. Kessler, *The End of Overeating*, Penguin, 2010

Pierre Pallardy, *Gut Instinct*, Rodale, 2007

Brian Wansink, *Mindless Eating*, Hay House, 2011

Acknowledgements

I would like to thank my agent Darley Anderson and his team, especially Sophie Gordon who believed in this book and Clare Wallace who is amazing.

I would also like to thank Anne Lawrance and Helen Stanton and everyone else at Little, Brown who has helped with this book.

Thanks also must go to all my family, my husband Michael and daughters Rosie and Molly, for their love and understanding.

About the Author

I am a therapist based in England with practices in Sheffield and London. I use a combination of therapies (Hypnotherapy, EFT and NLP) to help adults, teens and children with a wide range of issues.

I also run Hyp-Slim weight-loss courses. These workshops incorporate hypnosis along with all the techniques used in this book to help people lose weight naturally and permanently.

A number of years ago, B.C. (Before Children), I completed a PhD in chemistry and conducted research at various universities.

After having children I decided that a career change was in order. What I really wanted was to see a life coach, but at the time I couldn't afford one. So I did the next best thing, and trained to become one myself! This led me into a world of therapy and self-help that, as a sceptical scientist, I had avoided for years. But this world has completely changed my life – for the better. I hope that with *Diet Coach* as your guide, it will change yours too.

For more information, visit:

www.kimberlywillis.co.uk